The
DASH Diet
for Beginners

JOHN CHATHAM

CONTENTS

INTRODUCTION

It's no secret that the American diet is blamed today for more nutrition-related diseases and conditions than ever before. A high intake of calories, unhealthful fats, salt, and sugar is a big part of the problem, as is the low intake of fiber, vitamins, minerals, and healthful fats. The good news is that positive dietary change can be the first line of defense against everything from obesity to hypertension to type 2 diabetes and immune system disorders.

Several years ago, the National Institutes of Health (NIH) created the DASH diet as an answer to the rising incidence of high blood pressure and the health problems it causes. The diet was developed because changing your eating regimen can have an enormous effect on your blood pressure. Add regular, moderate exercise and you will experience a lifestyle change that can reduce or even reverse high blood pressure.

Before you cringe at the thought of boring, tasteless food and endless hours of exercise, be assured that the DASH diet includes a wide variety of all the foods and meals you enjoy most. It is not a severe, restrictive diet. It is a new way of preparing some of your favorite foods so that sodium is reduced but all the delicious flavor remains intact. You also don't need to spend so much time at the gym. This book will show you how to get moving, spend thirty minutes or less working out, and actually have fun doing it.

DASH Diet for Beginners isn't a harsh regimen; it's a way to enjoy your life and the foods you love while kick-starting your health and fitness. So read on with excitement, not dread. You'll love the choices you're about to make.

The DASH Diet Basics

$$\left(\textbf{1}\right)$$

WHAT IS THE DASH DIET?

The DASH diet is not so much a diet as it is a tool for creating a healthier lifestyle. It was created by the National Institutes of Health (NIH) as a way for people with high blood pressure to enjoy the foods they love while working to reduce or correct their hypertension.

The diet uses healthful food choices, along with more nutritious ways to prepare favorite dishes, to allow people to eat a varied, delicious, and balanced diet. This is not the type of diet to adopt for a number of weeks or months for the sole purpose of losing weight; rather, this is a new and healthier approach to food and eating.

Although it wasn't created as a weight-loss diet, the DASH diet often does result in weight loss. That weight loss is a huge benefit to those who either have high blood pressure or are at high risk of developing the disease. Obesity, or the condition of being excessively overweight (having a body mass index, or BMI, of 30 or greater), is one of the leading indicators of hypertension, and it also contributes to some of the conditions associated with high blood pressure, such as stroke and heart disease.

Sodium Reduction Guidelines

With the DASH diet, followers are given guidelines for both caloric intake and sodium consumption. The standard DASH diet allows up to 2,300 milligrams (mg) of sodium per day, while the low-sodium version allows up to 1,500 mg of sodium daily. This is in comparison to the typical American diet, which contains as much as 3,500 mg of sodium in an average day.

Increase Fiber Consumption

The DASH diet also recommends a higher fiber intake than is typical in most Americans' diets. The diet includes several servings of high-fiber vegetables, fruits, and grains each day, which not only help reduce blood pressure but also help you feel full and satisfied throughout the day.

In addition, the high-fiber content of the diet helps keep blood sugar levels steady and within safe ranges, and maximizes weight loss.

Focus on Healthful Fats

On the DASH diet, there is a very strong emphasis on getting plenty of healthful fats while reducing the intake of fats that aren't good for your health. Saturated and trans fats are kept to a minimum by switching out processed and fast foods for whole foods like low-fat dairy, lean meats, and omega-3–rich fish, seafood, nuts, and seeds.

These healthier fat choices help increase overall health by lowering LDL cholesterol and raising HDL cholesterol. This is important for individuals with high blood pressure, as heart disease is one of the more dangerous risks involved in hypertension.

Reduce Alcohol and Caffeine Consumption

Although alcohol, coffee, tea, and sodas are not strictly forbidden, they are limited, as they provide no nutrition, can elevate blood pressure, and are often loaded with sugar. Because type 2 diabetes and metabolic syndrome often accompany high blood pressure, the DASH guidelines limit sugary foods to just five servings per day. If you enjoy a glass of wine with dinner or an occasional cocktail, however, don't despair; you'll be able to continue enjoying them in moderation.

The same is true of your morning coffee, your afternoon tea, or your favorite afternoon soda. You can enjoy them as long as you're following the rest of the diet and exercise guidelines and are keeping your intake of these caffeinated drinks to the required healthful minimum.

A Healthful Intake of Vitamins and Minerals

The DASH diet's wide variety of fruits, vegetables, grains, and other whole foods ensures that you get enough of all the essential vitamins and minerals needed for good health. However, it also provides a healthful supply of minerals known to improve or reduce blood pressure, such as magnesium and potassium. You'll get a sufficient amount of these minerals by eating plenty of leafy greens, bananas, and legumes.

Your Caloric and Sodium Intake Is Customizable to You

On the standard DASH diet you can consume up to 2,300 mg of sodium per day; the lower sodium DASH diet allows up to 1,500 mg of sodium per day. You can also choose to eat a diet that provides anywhere from 1,500-3,100 calories per day. Which of these calorie and sodium limits you choose and how you combine them depends entirely upon your needs.

You (and your doctor, if you're working with one) can choose a lower calorie diet if you are overweight, or a higher calorie diet if you're very active or just want to maintain your current weight. You can choose a higher sodium intake if you don't currently have high blood pressure but want to prevent it in the future. You can choose the lower sodium level if you have high blood pressure now or you're at high risk for developing it due to being overweight or to your family history.

The different sodium and calorie plans can be combined in any way that best suits your current health and your goals.

The History of the DASH Diet

In 1992, the NIH funded research into a dietary answer to the growing incidence of high blood pressure in the United States. The goal was a nutritional plan that could reduce or improve hypertension.

The National Heart, Lung, and Blood Institute (NHLBI), which is a branch of the NIH, took on this research project, with the help of some of the most respected and advanced medical research institutions in the United States. Included were Johns Hopkins University, Brigham and Women's Hospital, Kaiser Permanente Center for Health Research, Duke University Medical Center, and Pennington Biomedical Research Center.

These five institutes, along with the NHLBI, conducted the most exhaustive research on high blood pressure that has ever been done in this country. The information collected by this group of researchers over the course of several years resulted in the creation of the Dietary Approaches to Stop Hypertension diet, or the DASH diet.

The DASH diet has since been widely recognized as one of the healthiest diets to follow. In 2012, the new Dietary Guidelines for Americans recommended the DASH diet for everyone, including kids and elderly people, regardless of whether or not they had high blood pressure. In fact, the new MyPlate dietary guidelines (which replaced the old food pyramid) are based largely on the DASH diet guidelines.

The Science Behind the DASH Diet

During the course of the research into the problems of high blood pressure and how nutrition can alleviate or improve them, several teams of physicians, nurses, and statistics experts worked with the participating institutions to conduct numerous clinical trials at each of the facilities. More than eight thousand Americans were screened for this research, two-thirds of whom were individuals from high-risk groups, such as African Americans, people with family histories of high blood pressure, and those who were overweight. Three different diets were given to the people participating in the study.

The Diets That Led to the Creation of the DASH Diet

The first diet, which was very close to the typical American diet, was considered the control. The only difference between this and the average American diet was the low-sodium intake of 1,500 milligrams per day. The purpose of this diet was to measure the effects of the lower sodium diet most often recommended by doctors to people with high blood pressure.

The second diet contained fewer snacks and more fruits and vegetables than the typical American diet. It was also significantly higher in fiber than the daily diet of the average American. The purpose of this diet was to observe the impact of a high-fiber diet on high blood pressure.

The third diet is the one that eventually became the DASH diet. Like the second diet, it was high in fiber, fruits, and vegetables. It was also low in saturated fats and high in minerals such as potassium and magnesium, which were thought to improve high blood pressure. However, the sodium intake allowed on this diet was 3,000 milligrams per day. The reason for this high quantity of sodium is that researchers wanted to see if making nutritional changes other than reduced sodium would have a positive impact on high blood pressure.

Exhaustive Study, Exciting Results

Two separate trials were conducted using these diets. In both trials, each group was placed on the first diet for three weeks, and their blood pressure, symptoms, and urine were monitored. After three weeks, four hundred participants were selected to continue in the trial on one of the three diets.

The data from the first trial showed that the low-sodium control diet did help lower the blood pressure of the participants. The DASH diet also helped, but not to a desirable degree. So in the second trial, the DASH diet was redesigned to include the lower sodium intake.

At the conclusion of the second study, the control diet was still showing an improvement in blood pressure, but the new DASH diet produced considerably better results, lowering blood pressure to a far more significant degree.

In fact, researchers found that after just thirty days on the new DASH diet, blood pressure was reduced by an average of 8.9/4.5 mm Hg (systolic/diastolic) in people who were considered at risk of high blood pressure, and by an average of 11.5/5.7 mm Hg in people already diagnosed with hypertension.

Not only that, but researchers also discovered that the new DASH diet lowered bad cholesterol and reduced body fat—in particular, dangerous abdominal fat. Researchers credit the low sugar intake for these benefits, since reducing sugar helps improve insulin sensitivity and promote fat loss.

Due to the results of this research, the DASH diet has become a highly recommended approach to eating for anyone, but especially for those concerned about high blood pressure.

THE HEALTH BENEFITS OF THE DASH DIET

Although the DASH diet was created primarily to reduce hypertension, the health benefits of the diet go far beyond lowering high blood pressure. As a result, the DASH diet is widely recommended by health organizations and physicians for many different types of people, for many reasons.

Although lowering high blood pressure or avoiding hypertension altogether are the main purposes of the DASH diet, those benefits are just the beginning of what the DASH diet can do for you.

The DASH Diet Lowers Blood Pressure

As discussed in the previous chapter, the final version of the DASH diet proved to be highly effective in lowering high blood pressure. The success of the diet in lowering high blood pressure is due to the low-sodium content and the increased fiber of the diet, as well as the intake of specific nutrients such as potassium and magnesium.

Not only is the DASH diet effective in lowering blood pressure, its effects are almost immediate. The Mayo Clinic, one of the facilities that participated in the study, had this to say about the fast results of following the DASH diet:

> *By following the DASH diet, you may be able to reduce your blood pressure by a few points in just two weeks. Over time, your blood pressure could drop by eight to fourteen points, which can make a significant difference in your health risks. (Nelson and Zeratsky, 2010)*

Obviously, the DASH diet is ideal for anyone who has high blood pressure or who may be at high risk of developing hypertension due to their weight, lifestyle, family medical history, or race.

The DASH Diet Can Prevent or Reverse Metabolic Syndrome or Prediabetes

Metabolic syndrome is often called "prediabetes" because it's considered a precursor to developing type 2 diabetes. However, it's not a condition in and of itself, but a collection of diagnostic indicators that include obesity, an excess of abdominal fat, a lack of sensitivity to insulin, high triglycerides and HDL cholesterol, and high fasting blood sugar levels.

The DASH diet is considered an excellent way of eating for those with metabolic syndrome for several reasons. Because the diet is very low in sugar, following the diet will increase your sensitivity to insulin and help correct both excess abdominal fat storage and high blood sugar. The low intake of unhealthful fats, combined with an increased intake of those fats that are good for you, will help lower HDL cholesterol and triglycerides. Last, because of the weight-loss benefit of the diet (if you choose a lower-calorie plan), excess weight and abdominal fat associated with metabolic syndrome are addressed.

The DASH Diet and Type 2 Diabetes

U.S. News & World Report rated the DASH diet as the best diet for people who either have type 2 diabetes or are at high risk of developing it.

The foods and guidelines of the DASH diet are highly beneficial for those with type 2 diabetes for the same reasons that it's so well regarded for reversing metabolic syndrome. Nuts can help to steady blood sugar and aid glucose control in diabetics, and the high-fiber nature of the diet also helps slow the absorption of sugar into the bloodstream.

One of the most important benefits to those with type 2 diabetes (or a high risk of developing it) is weight loss. Excess body fat, especially stored abdominal fat, is one of the biggest factors in a lack of insulin sensitivity. It also increases the risk of developing heart disease—a risk that diabetics already face.

The DASH Diet and Heart Disease

The American Heart Association (AHA) is one of the biggest supporters of the DASH diet.

In addition to being easy to follow, delicious and varied, the DASH eating plan is proven effective. According to one study, it reduced systolic and diastolic blood pressure by 5.5 and 3.0 mm Hg compared to the control diet (what the average American eats). The study showed that the DASH eating plan lowered blood pressure in virtually all subgroups defined by race, sex, age, body mass index, education, income, physical activity level, alcohol intake and hypertension status. It was particularly effective in African Americans and those diagnosed with hypertension. (AHA, 2012)

People with type 2 diabetes, metabolic syndrome, and high blood pressure face a much higher risk of developing heart disease. Since the DASH diet can improve or prevent those conditions, it's also an excellent diet for the prevention of heart disease.

Heart disease is the leading cause of death in America, and much of the incidence of heart disease can be traced back to an unhealthful diet. The typical American diet is low in fiber and healthful fats, and far too high in calories, unhealthful fats, and processed foods. This is why the DASH diet has gained the support of AHA, because it includes all of the components of a heart-healthful diet.

The DASH Diet Improves Overall Health

The DASH diet is one that conforms to all of the most respected research on bettering your overall health and lowering risks of disease through nutrition. Losing weight on the DASH diet is a wonderful bonus, but don't forget the impact that the diet is having on your longevity and quality of life.

The DASH diet has been approved and endorsed by some of the foremost medical experts in the country because it addresses so many critical health concerns. If you're going on the DASH diet in order to lose weight, it's important to remember that weight loss is just a happy side benefit of the diet. However, you should be even happier that your quality of life (and the length of your life) can be vastly improved!

Losing Weight on the DASH Diet

The DASH diet's food and guidelines include so many of the things that are known to be effective for safe, lasting weight loss that it's ideal for anyone trying to lose weight, regardless of whether they have high blood pressure.

Because the DASH diet is such a healthful one, you can and should follow it for your lifetime. It is not a quick-fix diet that is unhealthful for your body or unsafe to continue for an extended period of time. This means that while you're enjoying your weight loss, you can feel good about what you're doing both for your body and your health. When you reach your weight-loss goal, you won't just be slimmer—you'll be healthier.

There are three things that make the DASH diet especially good for weight loss, aside from watching calories: a focus on eating healthful fats/omitting unhealthful fats, increased fiber intake, and a high intake of vitamin C and other nutrients.

The DASH Diet's Fat Profile

On the DASH diet, you'll be eating far less of the unhealthful fats that are typical in the average American diet. Trans fats and unhealthful saturated fats are strictly limited or even omitted, while healthful fats, such as plant-based saturated fats and omega-3 fats, are much higher than in the typical American diet. While this is great for your heart, it's also great for your waist.

The foods that are usually high in unhealthful fats, such as fast food and highly processed foods, are usually very high in calories and low in nutritional content. The DASH diet focuses on whole foods, giving you the satisfaction and nutrition you need without all of the empty calories.

The DASH Diet's Fiber Profile

A high-fiber diet is not only great for your health but also great for your weight. The DASH diet is loaded with delicious foods that are high in both soluble and insoluble fiber. This helps you to feel satisfied, improves your digestion, and slows the absorption of dietary fat and sugar.

This means less new stored fat in the abdominal area and fewer blood sugar spikes (and the attending cravings for carbs and junk foods).

The DASH Diet's Vitamin C Profile

Because the DASH diet is filled with delicious and nutrient-rich fresh fruits and vegetables, you'll be getting plenty of essential vitamins and minerals, as well as a wide range of antioxidants. One of the most important to your weight-loss efforts is vitamin C.

Vitamin C has been shown over recent years to be an essential tool in eliminating stored fat and preventing hormonal reactions that promote the storage of fat in the abdominal area.

Vitamin C is depleted by many things, but daily stress is one of the biggest culprits. When your vitamin C levels are too low, it can signal to your brain that you're under stress, which then results in the release of the stress hormone cortisol. Cortisol's job is to store fat in the abdominal area as a kind if insurance against famine. While stress doesn't necessarily equal famine the way it did in the past, your body perceives it the same way.

When you reduce the stress in your life, you also reduce the amount of cortisol being released into your bloodstream. It's not possible for the average person to eliminate all stress, but getting enough vitamin C can counter its effects and correct the levels of cortisol being released. Less cortisol means less new stored fat, but it also alerts your body to the fact that you no longer need all the stored fat you already have! Vitamin C plays an important role at this point, too.

Vitamin C is a primary component of a naturally occurring compound called L-carnitine. L-carnitine is sometimes called the fat-transport compound, because it's responsible for carrying stored fat to where the body can convert it into glucose and burn it as energy.

Our bodies make L-carnitine, but they require a healthful supply of vitamin C to do so. Our bodies prioritize the use of the vitamin C in our systems at any given time. The first priority is to use it to fight infection and rebuild cells. Whatever is leftover can be used for building L-carnitine.

The problem is that vitamin C is a soluble vitamin; our bodies flush most of it out with our urine and store only a very small supply. This is why getting plenty of vitamin C on a daily basis is so essential to losing body fat. The DASH diet addresses this problem by being high in the fresh fruits and vegetables that have the greatest vitamin C content. Not only will you be able to burn stored fat, you'll also be giving your immune system the boost it needs.

The DASH diet uses these factors to help you lose weight safely, comfortably, and in a way that benefits your overall health. It also uses a sane, but entirely livable calorie intake to help you toward your goals. This portion of the DASH diet is completely customizable to you, your goals, and your caloric needs. The next chapter will show you how to choose the caloric option that is best for you, so you can be on your way to meeting your weight-loss goals without starving yourself or feeling deprived.

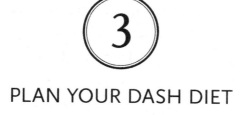

PLAN YOUR DASH DIET

Just as with any successful venture, there are a few steps that you need to take in order to make your DASH diet as painless as possible. By the time you finish this book, you're going to have a great starting point and a well-defined map to set you off on your path to health and fitness.

Throughout the following pages, you're going to figure out exactly where you stand and what you need to do in order to reach your personal goals. This chapter will:

- Show you how to calculate your *body mass index* (BMI) and how to use it to set your end goal
- Explain how to use your *basal metabolic rate* (BMR) and your BMI to work out your caloric needs
- Teach you how to use these figures along with the meal plan and your own tastes to help you stay on course and meet your goals

The end of this chapter will discuss common pitfalls and how you can avoid them in order to ensure success. It's going to take some effort and some good decision making on your part, but if you stick with it, you're going to love the end result—a healthier, leaner you!

Starting Your DASH Diet

Before you take a single step toward the grocery store or the gym, you need to figure out exactly where your body is starting from. After all, every good journey starts somewhere, right? You're going to need a log book to keep track of your progress. There are a few numbers that you're going to need in order to determine the condition of your body right now.

- **Weight:** Regardless of what many people believe, this isn't the best indicator of health or fitness, but it's still a necessary component to help you set your goals. Weigh yourself first thing in the morning with an empty bladder before you eat anything, and record the number in your log book.
- **Body Mass Index (BMI):** This is a much more accurate reflection of your current state because it measures your level of body fat, which is, after all, what you're trying to change. There are a couple of ways to do this. You can either buy a tool that gauges your BMI based upon your stats and measurements, or you can measure yourself and use an online calculator, such as the one you'll find at http://www.linear-software.com/online.html.

If you use a tape measure, make sure the tape is snug against your skin but not pulled so tight that it cuts into your flesh—you want an accurate measurement.

If you're a woman, you'll need to measure your waist, hips, and neck at their narrowest points, and your height. If you're a man, measure your neck, your stomach just below your navel, and your height.

Go to the online calculator and choose your gender, then choose the "tape" method of calculation. Enter your numbers, and then click the "calculate" button. Enter this number in your log book under your starting measurements.

- *Basal Metabolic Rate (BMR):* This is the amount of calories that you burn per day at rest. It is a much more accurate formula than simply using your body weight, because your gender, age, and height play a huge role in how your body burns calories. Here's how you figure it:

- **Women:** BMR = 655 + (4.35 x weight in pounds) + (4.7 x height in inches) − (4.7 x age in years)

- **Men:** BMR = 66 + (6.23 x weight in pounds) + (12.7 x height in inches) − (6.8 x age in years)

This isn't an exact calculation, because it doesn't take your BMI into consideration, and muscle burns more calories than fat, so if you're leaner, you'd burn more calories than a person who had a higher percentage of body fat, even if both of you were the exact same height, weight, and age. Still, your BMR is an excellent tool to use. Next you need to factor in your activity level in order to get a more accurate idea of how many calories you're actually burning. To do this, use the following guidelines.

- Sedentary (little or no exercise):
  Calorie Calculation = BMR x 1.2

- Mildly active (exercise 1–3 days per week):
  Calorie Calculation = BMR x 1.375

- Moderately active (exercise 3–5 days per week):
  Calorie Calculation = BMR x 1.55

- Very active (exercise 6–7 days per week):
  Calorie Calculation = BMR x 1.725

- Extremely active (exercise and physical job or double training daily):
  Calorie Calculation = BMR x 1.9

This is the number of calories that you burn on a daily basis. Since weight loss is a numbers game, the goal is to increase the amount of calories that you burn, while decreasing the number of calories that you consume, in order to lose weight.

Since one pound is equivalent to 3,500 calories, you need to deduct 500 calories per day in order to lose one pound per week. If you want to lose two pounds per week, you'd need to consume 1,000 calories less per day. You could also burn that many more calories per day in order to see the same results. Since it's not recommended that you consume less than 1,500 calories per day if you are a woman, or 1,800 calories per day if you are a man, the best plan is to eat less and exercise more.

Monitor Your Numbers Closely, but Not Too Closely

Because you are going to be using your weight, BMI, and BMR to map out your program, remember that these numbers change. Weighing and measuring yourself daily can be discouraging, but you need to do so at least once per week so that you can maintain steady progress. As you lose fat, gain muscle, and increase your activity levels, your caloric needs are going to change, so keep an eye on them, and adjust as necessary.

Ten Tips for Getting Started

Changing your lifestyle may not be easy, but keeping your eye on the end goal will help. Getting through the first couple of weeks will be your biggest challenge. After that, you will have established new eating and exercise habits, and it will simply be a way of life for you. Following these tips can help you get off to a quick start and feel great as you improve your health, lose weight, and create a better lifestyle.

1. Plan to Cook at Home in the Beginning

One of the hardest things about changing your eating habits is giving up those French fries and decadent sauces. To help keep you on the straight and narrow, it may be better to avoid restaurants altogether until you see some concrete results that will help strengthen your resolve.

2. Lay Off Salt and Other High-Calorie, Nutrient-Poor Condiments

There are plenty of great herbs and seasonings that you can use to add flavor to your food. If you're a salt addict, switch to a salt substitute, such as the aptly named Mrs. Dash. This is not only important from a weight-loss perspective; it will also help if you have high blood pressure, heart disease, or kidney problems.

3. Get Rid of Junk in the Pantry

When you are first starting out, it's best to operate under the out-of-sight, out-of-mind theory. It's going to be much more difficult to avoid chips, candy, soda, and processed foods if they are staring you in the face every time you open the pantry. Get rid of them, and replace them with fruits and veggies.

4. Exercise in the Morning

Until you get into the habit of exercising regularly, it's best to get it out of the way early. That way, things can't come up that will give you an excuse to avoid it. Once exercise is a regular part of your life, you can adapt your schedule if you want to.

5. Nip Emotional Eating in the Bud

Many people eat more than they need to, for various reasons. You may be bored, stressed, or just in the habit of heading to the fridge whenever you pass the kitchen, but you need to break that habit. Engage in behaviors that aren't compatible with snacking, such as exercising, calling a friend on the phone, or cleaning house. Exercise releases endorphins that will relieve stress and get you through that urge to eat.

6. Plan for Eating Situations

There are simply times when food is part of life. This may be football games, movies, or just getting through that 2:00 p.m. energy crash. If you plan for them in advance by taking healthful snacks or deciding to go for a walk instead of heading to the office vending machine, you won't sabotage your hard work.

7. Find Healthful Foods That You Like

Just because broccoli is part of a snack or meal on your meal plan, don't feel that you have to eat it if you don't like it. Find a suitable replacement that you *do* like, because forcing yourself to eat things that you don't like is a recipe for failure. Eating healthful meals is difficult enough; fill your diet with foods you love, or you won't be able to stick with it.

8. Drink Water!

Drinking plenty of water is important for more reasons than one. First, it will help you feel full, making it easier to pass on those opportunities to eat when you're not hungry. Water also helps your body flush out fat and toxins so that you lose fat and become healthier faster. To calculate how much water you need, divide your current weight in half, and convert that to ounces. In other words, if you weigh two hundred pounds, you should drink one hundred ounces of water per day.

9. Get a Friend on Board

Sticking with a diet and exercise plan is much easier if you have company. You can support each other, and it's nice to have someone you care about to discuss your challenges and successes with. At the very least, let your family know how important this is to you, so they can be there to offer support when you need it.

10. Keep a "Food and Feelings" Journal

Writing down your feelings after exercising, and recording how you feel when you succeed is a great way to stay motivated. Whether you opt for an apple instead of apple pie, or you lose an inch from your waist, write down how you feel about it. Then when you hit a rough patch, go back and read your thoughts—and discover your own personal cheering section!

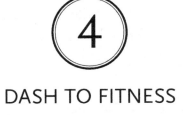

DASH TO FITNESS

Fitting enough exercise into your daily life is as essential to good health as eating the right foods. Whether you're trying to lose weight, lower your blood pressure, or reverse metabolic syndrome, exercise is key to achieving your goals.

Moderate, regular exercise lowers blood pressure, helps to build your cardiovascular health, supports a healthful metabolism, and promotes the loss of fat stored on the body. These are all key elements to fighting hypertension, heart disease, and metabolic syndrome.

If your goal is also to lose weight, you need exercise to do it well. Cutting calories alone is a difficult way to lose weight. For instance, if you want to lose one pound of fat per week, you'll need to cut 500 calories a day from your diet, since one pound of fat equals 3,500 calories. It's much easier to cut 250 calories a day, and burn another 250 calories through a short session of moderate exercise. Exercise also speeds up your metabolism, which means you'll burn more calories throughout the day.

You need both cardio exercise and strength training or resistance exercise for optimum health. Cardio will burn calories and improve your heart and lung health. Strength training will build lean muscle (which also speeds your metabolism), improve bone strength and density, and reshape your body as you lose weight.

The seven-day workout plan includes both cardio and resistance or strength-training workouts. This plan is designed for exercise beginners, but you can easily adjust it to suit your needs if you've been working out regularly and are reasonably fit. It's a simple plan, but that makes it more flexible. You can adjust it as you become more fit.

The Seven-Day Workout Plan

This plan is designed to be a safe and workable program, even for those who are significantly overweight or have been sedentary for quite some time. However, it's very important that you talk with your doctor before starting any exercise program!

Following this plan for the first month of your diet will help ease you safely into working out, while still giving you plenty of cardiovascular and calorie-burning benefits and helping you build some lean muscle.

Once you've been on the program for a month or so (or if you're starting out more advanced), you can easily increase the effectiveness of your cardio by lengthening the sessions, increasing your pace, or kicking up the intensity (such as walking uphill or swimming the butterfly stroke).

You can tweak your resistance-training sessions by adding dumbbells or weight machines to your program. This will build lean muscle faster and speed up the process of transforming your body.

Feel free to switch back and forth between cardio exercises. You can walk one week and swim the next, or walk Monday, swim Wednesday, and cycle Friday. The more variety you have, the less chance that your body will adapt too quickly and begin to plateau.

- **MONDAY:** Thirty minutes of moderate cardio. Choose walking (outdoors or on a treadmill), cycling (on a bicycle or stationary bike), or swimming. A moderate pace is one at which you can talk with some effort.

- **TUESDAY:** Twenty minutes of body-weight resistance exercises, such as squats, lunges, push-ups, and pull-ups.

- **WEDNESDAY:** Thirty minutes of moderate cardio, either walking, cycling, or swimming.

- **THURSDAY:** Twenty minutes of body-weight resistance exercises.

- **FRIDAY:** Thirty minutes of moderate cardio.

- **SATURDAY:** Twenty minutes of body-weight resistance exercises.

- **FREE DAY!** If you like, do another session of cardio. Otherwise, take the day off.

WHAT'S ON THE DASH DIET PLATE?

The first thing people wonder when undertaking a new diet is, "What do I get to eat?" The happy news with the DASH diet is that you get to eat quite a lot! The DASH diet is filled with plenty of delicious and filling, whole foods, such as fruits, vegetables, whole grains, seafood, poultry, and lean meats. Although sweets are limited, you can enjoy some delicious and decadent desserts on the diet as well. You won't feel hungry or deprived on the DASH diet, which is one of the things that makes it so effective.

Planning Your Daily Meals

One of the goals of the DASH diet is to steady or correct blood sugar spikes and drops that leave you feeling fatigued, foggy, and moody, and can also lead to metabolic syndrome or type 2 diabetes.

For that reason, eat as early as possible upon rising and then space out your meals and snacks so that you're eating at least every two to three hours. This will keep your blood sugar steady, give you the energy you need to get through your day, and help you avoid the pitfalls of hunger and carb cravings.

In the interests of healthful blood-sugar levels (as well as losing weight), you'll also want to focus on low-glycemic varieties of fruits and vegetables first, then sprinkle your diet with moderate- to high-glycemic varieties if some of them are your favorites. Just use moderation and don't consume too many of them in one day, as this will raise blood sugar and can slow the rate at which your body adjusts to a lower sugar intake. In the DASH Diet Foods List later in this chapter, you'll see those foods broken down into their respective categories.

There's absolutely nothing wrong with taking some of your fruits, vegetables, and other foods from breakfast, lunch, or dinner, and repurposing them as snacks. Actually, the more often you enjoy a small, healthful snack, the better. This could be something as simple as an apple, or more like a mini-meal, with a serving of protein and a fresh vegetable or whole grain on the side.

One thing important to bear in mind as you plan your diet is that you choose several servings of foods rich in potassium, magnesium, and calcium. These are the micronutrients that the DASH studies showed to be so effective in lowering blood pressure.

What about Salt?

The DASH diet recommends that you keep your sodium intake at or below 2,300 mg per day. If you have high blood pressure or are at risk of developing it, however, you may want to adopt the 1,500 mg per day plan. Eating whole foods, rather than restaurant or store-bought packaged foods, will go a long way toward reducing the sodium in your diet. You'll also want to pay close attention to the labels on products such as cereals, condiments, soups, breads, and other prepared foods, as they're often loaded with unexpected sodium.

The DASH Diet Foods List will help you choose foods that are lower in sodium, but you'll want to note your sodium intake in a small notebook if you're on a low-sodium plan.

The DASH Diet Foods List

Until you get accustomed to the DASH diet, you may want to make copies of this foods list to take with you to the grocery store. This will simplify your shopping and help you to plan your meals as you go.

Meats and Seafood

Allowed:

- All fish, especially salmon, haddock, mackerel, sardines, and other oily fish
- All shellfish
- Beef: lean steaks and roasts, and leanest possible ground meat
- Chicken, skinless
- Eggs
- Game birds
- Game meats
- Lamb: lean stew meat, steaks, and roasts
- Pork: lean steaks and roasts
- Turkey: skinless and ground breast
- Venison

Not Allowed:

- Bacon, except for low-sodium turkey bacon
- Jerky
- Packaged cold cuts and deli meats (use leftover homemade meats or low-sodium deli counter meats)
- Sausage

Dairy

Allowed:

- Almond milk
- Bleu cheese
- Cheddar cheese (reduced fat)
- Cottage cheese (low or nonfat)
- Cow's milk (skim or 1 percent)
- Cream cheese (reduced fat)
- Feta cheese
- Greek yogurt
- Margarine or butter substitute
- Mozzarella cheese
- Parmesan cheese (high sodium, so limit quantities)
- Provolone cheese (reduced fat)
- Regular yogurt (low or nonfat)
- Ricotta cheese (reduced fat)
- Roquefort cheese
- Soy milk
- Sour cream (reduced or nonfat)
- Swiss cheese

Not Allowed:

- Any full-fat dairy products
- Butter
- Cream

Low-Glycemic Vegetables

(Eat as much as you like.)

Allowed:

- Artichokes
- Arugula
- Asparagus
- Avocados
- Bell peppers
- Broccoli
- Brussels sprouts
- Cabbages
- Cauliflowers
- Celery
- Collard greens
- Cucumbers
- Eggplants
- Green beans
- Kale
- Lettuce, preferably romaine or dark leafy varieties
- Mushrooms
- Mustard greens
- Onions
- Radishes
- Snow peas
- Spinach
- Swiss chard
- Sprouts
- Summer squashes
- Turnip greens
- Zucchini

Higher Glycemic Vegetables

(Make these secondary choices.)

Allowed:

- Acorn squashes
- Butternut squashes
- Carrots
- Chickpeas
- English peas
- Spaghetti squashes
- Sweet potatoes
- Tomatoes

Not Allowed:

- Corn
- White potatoes

Lower Glycemic Fruits

(All fruits are allowed. Make these your primary choices.)

- Apples
- Apricots
- Bananas
- Blackberries
- Blueberries
- Cantaloupe
- Casaba melon
- Cranberries
- Grapes

- Guavas
- Honeydew melon
- Lemons
- Limes
- Nectarines
- Papayas
- Peaches
- Raspberries
- Rhubarb
- Strawberries
- Watermelons

Higher Glycemic Fruits

(Make these secondary choices.)

- Cherries
- Figs
- Grapefruits
- Kiwis
- Mangos
- Oranges
- Pears
- Plums
- Pumpkin
- Tangerines
- Watermelon

Fats

Allowed:

- Almonds
- Black walnuts
- Brazil nuts
- Canola oil
- Flaxseed oil
- Margarine or butter substitute
- Mayonnaise (low fat)
- Pecans
- Olives (low sodium)
- Olive oil
- Sesame seeds
- Sunflower seeds

Not Allowed:

- All other vegetable oils, including peanut oil and sesame oil

Grains

Allowed:

- Almond flour
- Barley
- Brown rice
- Coconut flour
- Wheat germ
- Whole-grain bread, preferably very dense
- Whole-grain, low-carb cold cereal

- Whole-grain, mixed-grain hot cereal
- Whole-grain pita
- Whole-grain steel-cut oats
- Whole-grain thin-style bagels
- Whole-grain thin-style English muffins
- Whole-grain tortillas
- Whole-wheat flour

Not Allowed:

- Corn meal
- Corn muffins or corn bread
- Instant or flavored oatmeal
- Sweetened cold cereals

Condiments, Seasonings, and Miscellaneous

Allowed:

- Agave nectar
- Almond butter
- Caesar dressing
- Coffee
- Dressings (low or no sodium)
- Flaxseed or flaxseed oil
- Herbs and spices
- Honey
- Hot sauce
- Mustard (except honey mustard)
- Peanut butter (in limited quantities)
- Preserves and jellies (low or no sugar)
- Psyllium husk

- Quinoa
- Salsa
- Sesame butter
- Sour or dill pickles
- Soy sauce (low sodium)
- Tea (hot or iced)
- Teriyaki sauce (low sodium)
- Tomato or spaghetti sauce (no sugar added)
- Vegetable, chicken, or beef broth (no or low sodium)
- Vinaigrette
- Whey or soy protein powder (no sugar added)

Not Allowed:

- Alfredo or cheese sauce (prepared)
- Gravies (prepared)
- Mayonnaise (full fat)
- Salad dressings (regular, commercial)
- Steak, barbecue, and other sauces (regular sodium)

Occasional Treats

(These are in addition to the dessert and snack recipes.)

- Dried fruits (preferably no sugar added)
- Frozen fruit bars (no sugar added)
- Fudge pops (fat free)
- Gelatin
- Ice cream (low fat)
- 1-ounce square dark chocolate
- Popsicles
- Pudding or pudding cups (fat free)
- Sorbet or sherbet

The DASH Diet Shopping Guide

Here are a few tips to making your grocery shopping easier and more nutritious.

Shop Around the Perimeter of the Store

Try to buy most of your food from the fresh food sections, which are normally placed around the perimeter of the store. This includes fresh fruits and vegetables, fresh meats, seafood, poultry, and fresh dairy products.

Read Labels

Don't assume that something is low in sodium just because it isn't salty—even some breakfast cereals and desserts are loaded with unwanted salt. Read the labels on everything from canned broth to spaghetti sauce to bread. Whenever possible, make your own versions of these convenience foods so that you can control the level of sodium.

Choose Meat and Seafood Wisely

Whenever you can, buy organic, grass-fed meats, or wild-caught seafood. They have more omega-3 fats and are usually free of hormones and preservatives. Always choose the leanest cuts of whatever you're buying, and trim visible fat after cooking.

Choose Low-Fat Dairy

Always select low-fat or nonfat dairy products so you'll still have fat servings left to choose from in other areas of your daily diet. Cheeses should be nonfat or part-skim; milk should be skim or 1 percent fat; and yogurt should be nonfat and low in sugar. Keep in mind that Greek yogurt will give you twice the protein of regular varieties.

DASH Diet Recipes & Meal Plans

- **Chapter 6**: Appetizer and Snack Recipes

- **Chapter 7**: Breakfast Recipes

- **Chapter 8**: Lunch Recipes

- **Chapter 9**: Dinner Recipes

- **Chapter 10**: Dessert Recipes

- **Chapter 11**: Seven-Day DASH Diet Meal Plan

APPETIZER AND SNACK RECIPES

Creamy Spinach Dip

This deliciously cheesy dip is wonderful served warm with some crusty bread or used as a tasty topping for sliced peppers, cucumbers, and tomatoes. This party-sized batch will be a hit with your guests, and they'll never know it's a DASH recipe.

- 3 (12-ounce) packages frozen chopped spinach, thawed and well drained
- 2 teaspoons freshly ground pepper
- 2 cloves fresh garlic, crushed
- 2 tablespoons fresh parsley, chopped
- 1 tablespoon fresh basil, chopped
- 1 (15-ounce) can Great Northern beans, well drained
- 2 tablespoons Parmesan cheese
- 1/2 cup low-fat sour cream

Preheat oven to 350 degrees.

In a medium-sized mixing bowl, combine spinach, pepper, garlic, parsley, and basil, and stir until well blended.

Stir in beans, Parmesan cheese, and sour cream until well combined, then pour into a shallow baking dish. Bake for 20-30 minutes or until bubbly.

Makes about 8 (1/2-cup) servings.

Calories: 95

Sodium: 70 mg

Creamy Kale Soup

Kale is one of the most nutrient-packed greens you can eat and has a unique, almost nutty flavor. This soup is a great starter for a fall or winter meal and also makes a nice light lunch or snack. The homemade croutons take just a few minutes and far surpass any store-bought versions.

For the herbed croutons:
- 2 tablespoons olive oil
- 1 teaspoon garlic powder
- 1 tablespoon fresh parsley, chopped
- 1 tablespoon fresh thyme, chopped
- 2 cups day-old whole-grain baguette or other crusty bread

For the soup:
- 1 tablespoon olive oil
- 1 small white onion, chopped
- 1 clove fresh garlic, crushed
- 1 tablespoon fresh thyme, chopped
- 2 cups new red potatoes, peeled and diced
- 1/4 teaspoon salt substitute
- 1/4 teaspoon freshly ground pepper
- 6 cups fresh kale, trimmed
- 4 cups low-sodium vegetable broth or stock

To make the herbed croutons:
Preheat oven to 350 degrees.

In a large bowl, combine olive oil, garlic powder, and herbs, then toss bread cubes to coat well. Do this fairly quickly so cubes don't become soaked.

Pour croutons onto a foil-lined baking sheet, and bake for about 10 minutes or just until golden and crisp. Set aside to cool.

To make the soup:
Heat olive oil in a large, heavy saucepan over medium heat. Add onion, garlic, and thyme, and sauté until onions are transparent (about 7-8 minutes).

Add potatoes, salt substitute, and freshly ground pepper, stirring well, then cover and let sauté another for 10-12 minutes or until potatoes are nearly tender.

Add kale and sauté uncovered for 5 minutes, then add vegetable broth, cover, and let simmer for another 5-7 minutes, until kale is tender but still bright green.

Transfer half of the soup to a blender or food processor and blend until smooth. Add back to the saucepan and stir well.

To serve, ladle into soup bowls and top with croutons.

Makes 6 servings.
Calories: 170
Sodium: 285 mg

Spinach-Stuffed Portobello Mushrooms

This is a great appetizer to serve when you have company, as it's easily made ahead (just broil at the last minute) and is equally enjoyable served room temperature or fresh from the broiler.

- 2 teaspoons olive oil, divided
- 2 cloves fresh garlic, crushed
- 1 tablespoon fresh tarragon, chopped
- 1/2 teaspoon freshly ground pepper
- 1 cup frozen chopped spinach, thawed and very well drained
- 4 large portobello mushroom stems, chopped
- 4 large portobello mushrooms caps
- 4 teaspoons grated Parmesan cheese

In a large, heavy skillet, heat 1 teaspoon olive oil over medium-high heat. Add garlic, tarragon, and freshly ground pepper, and sauté for 1 minute.

Add spinach and mushroom stems to pan, and sauté for 3-4 minutes, or until stems are slightly tender. Remove to a bowl.

Add remaining olive oil to pan, and once heated, place mushroom caps in pan with grill side up. Sauté without turning for 3 minutes, turn over, then cover and turn heat to low.

Sauté for another 2 minutes.

Remove caps to a foil-lined baking sheet, grill side up. Divide spinach mixture between them, top with Parmesan cheese, and place on rack 6 inches from broiler. Broil for 3-4 minutes.

Makes 2 servings.

Calories: 90

Sodium: 120 mg

Chewy Cranberry-Apricot Bars

This delicious bar is great for a quick snack, a light dessert, or even an on-the-go breakfast. It's loaded with fiber, and the dried fruits provide plenty of vitamins and minerals.

- Canola oil spray
- 2 cups uncooked, multigrain hot cereal
- 1 cup bran flakes
- 1/2 cup chopped walnuts
- 1/2 cup dried apricots, chopped
- 1/2 cup dried cranberries
- 1/2 cup dry skim milk powder
- 3/4 cup honey
- 3/4 cup unsalted almond butter
- 1 tablespoon canola oil
- 1 tablespoon vanilla

Preheat oven to 325 degrees.

Lightly coat a 9 x 13–inch pan with canola oil spray.

In a large bowl, combine cereal, bran flakes, walnuts, dried apricots, dried cranberries, and dry milk powder.

In a small, nonstick saucepan, combine honey, almond butter, and canola oil, and cook over medium-low heat, stirring frequently. When mixture begins to bubble, remove pan from heat, and stir in vanilla.

Pour the hot mixture over the cereal and fruit mixture, and stir until completely incorporated.

Use a spatula or wooden spoon to spread the mixture evenly into the baking pan, and pat it down well.

Bake for 20 minutes, then cool on a rack for 20 minutes before cutting into 12 snack-sized bars. Serve warm or room temperature, and store in an airtight container.

Makes 12 servings.
Calories: 175
Sodium: 28 mg

Crispy Kale Chips

Potato chips and other salty snacks are some of the first foods people fear they'll crave when someone mentions a low-sodium diet. With these deliciously different kale chips, you can have a salty chip-like snack in just minutes, but they're loaded with vitamins and flavor, not fat and salt.

- 1 bunch (about 4 cups) fresh kale
- 1 tablespoon olive oil
- 1 teaspoon salt substitute

Preheat oven to 275 degrees.

Remove the toughest ribs from the kale leaves, then bunch leaves together and cut into approximately 3-inch pieces.

Place kale onto a large, rimmed cookie sheet, drizzle with olive oil, and toss to coat well.

Sprinkle with salt substitute, toss again, and spread out as close to a single layer as possible.

Bake for 12 minutes, turn each kale chip over with tongs, and bake for another 10 minutes.

These are best eaten immediately.

Makes 4 servings.
Calories: 60
Sodium: 26 mg

Tropical Salsa

This deliciously different salsa has a wonderful blend of sweet and spicy flavors, with no salt added, freeing you up to enjoy it with some low-sodium tortilla or pita chips, or just use it on your favorite taco or burrito.

- 4 plum tomatoes, diced
- 1 medium mango, barely ripe, diced
- 1 medium, sweet white onion, chopped
- 1 small, fresh jalapeño pepper, chopped
- 2 cloves fresh garlic, crushed
- 1/4 cup fresh cilantro, chopped
- 1/4 cup fresh parsley, chopped
- 1 teaspoon cumin
- 1/4 teaspoon freshly ground pepper
- Juice and zest of 1 large lime

In a medium-sized bowl, combine tomatoes, mango, onion, jalapeño, and garlic, stirring until well blended.

Add fresh herbs, cumin, and freshly ground pepper, and stir well. Add lime zest, and stir again, then add lime juice, and stir once more. Allow to rest at room temperature for about 1 hour before serving, or refrigerate for up to 2 days before eating.

Note: If you're sensitive to hot peppers, remove and discard the pepper's inner core and seeds before chopping. This will reduce the fiery impact of the jalapeño, but will leave you plenty of flavor. Just be careful not to touch your face' or eyes after handling the inside of the pepper—or wear a rubber glove!

Makes 4 servings.
Calories: 55
Sodium: 8 mg

Pick-Me-Up Yogurt Smoothie

Your busy schedule might not allow for a sit-down snack, but it does leave you in need of some extra energy. This fast smoothie has the protein and fruit to see you through the rest of your day.

- 1 (6-ounce) container of peach or mango Greek yogurt
- 1/2 cup unsweetened pineapple chunks
- 1/4 cup plain almond milk
- 6-8 ice cubes

In a blender, combine yogurt, pineapple, and almond milk, and blend just until smooth. Add ice cubes and blend on high until thick and creamy. Serve immediately.

Makes 1 large smoothie.

Calories: 215

Sodium: 112 mg

Quick Tomato and Mozzarella Mini-Tarts

This recipe uses a muffin tin and ordinary whole-wheat bread to create elegantly rustic mini-tarts that are pretty and tasty enough for company, but take only minutes to make. As a bonus, each serving packs 254 mg of potassium!

- 1 teaspoon olive oil
- 8 slices low-sodium, whole-wheat bread
- 2 large tomatoes, diced
- 1 cup shredded low-fat mozzarella cheese
- 1/2 teaspoon freshly ground pepper
- 2 tablespoons fresh basil, chopped
- 2 tablespoons fresh oregano, chopped

Preheat oven to 350 degrees.

Rub insides and edges of an 8-cup muffin tin with olive oil.

On a cutting board, remove crusts from bread, and use a rolling pin or heavy glass to flatten each slice. Press 1 slice into each muffin cup, using your fingers to press down and mold to the sides. Trim excess roughly to leave a rustic-looking edge.

In a small bowl, combine tomatoes and mozzarella, then add freshly ground pepper and toss. Divide mixture between the muffin cups.

In the same bowl, combine basil and oregano well, then sprinkle over each cup.

Bake for 12-14 minutes or until the cheese is bubbly. Let cool for 10 minutes before removing from muffin tin. Serve warm or at room temperature.

Makes 4 servings.
Calories: 294
Sodium: 520 mg

BREAKFAST RECIPES

Veggie Scramble

This recipe is loaded with so many fresh veggies that you get quite a few servings packed into just one meal. If you prefer, you can use whole eggs instead of egg whites for the scramble. There's so much flavor here that you'll never miss the typical fat- and sodium-dense omelet.

- 1 teaspoon olive oil
- 1/2 large red bell pepper, julienned
- 1/2 large yellow pepper, julienned
- 1 small sweet white onion, chopped
- 1 clove garlic, crushed
- 6 white button mushrooms, sliced
- 1/2 teaspoon salt substitute
- 1/2 teaspoon freshly ground pepper
- 6 egg whites
- 1/4 cup fresh parsley, chopped

In a large, heavy skillet, heat olive oil over medium-high heat.

Add peppers, onion, and garlic, and sauté for about 5 minutes until veggies are tender-crisp. Add mushrooms and sauté for 2 more minutes.

Add salt substitute and freshly ground pepper to the egg whites, and pour into skillet. Sauté just until eggs are set. Garnish with fresh parsley, and serve alone or over a slice of whole-grain toast.

Makes 2 servings.

Calories: 129

Sodium: 170 mg

Better-Than-a-Latte Smoothie

There's nothing like a fresh, creamy latte, unless it's this more filling and nutritious alternative. Save time and money by making your own frappe-type coffee drink, and you can count it as breakfast, too. If the smoothie isn't sweet enough, add just enough sugar to suit you.

- 1 (6-ounce) container vanilla Greek yogurt
- 1/2 cup vanilla almond milk
- 1/4 cup espresso, cooled to room temperature
- 6 ice cubes
- 1/4 teaspoon nutmeg or cinnamon

In a blender, combine yogurt, almond milk, and espresso until well blended. Add ice cubes and blend until thick and smooth. Pour into glass, then sprinkle with nutmeg or cinnamon.

Makes 1 large smoothie.

Calories: 112

Sodium: 187 mg

Toasted Oat and Fruit Parfait

It's a good idea to toast extra batches of oats and nuts on the weekend, then keep them in an airtight container to use throughout the week in recipes like this oat and fruit parfait. This recipe is not only delicious, it's loaded with protein and healthful fats that will power you through your busy mornings. It also contains a walloping 790 mg of potassium.

- 1 cup whole rolled oats, uncooked
- 1/2 cup black walnuts, chopped
- 1/4 cup raisins
- 2 teaspoons dark or light brown sugar
- 1 cup vanilla Greek yogurt
- 1/4 cup dried cranberries

In a large heavy skillet, toast oats, walnuts, raisins, and brown sugar over medium heat for 3-4 minutes. The mixture will become sticky. Remove from pan and set aside to cool.

Once oat mixture has cooled to room temperature, assemble alternate layers of oats, yogurt, and cranberries in 2 dessert glasses.

Makes 2 servings.

Calories: 575

Sodium: 52 mg

Blueberry and Quinoa Cereal

Quinoa is often mistaken for a grain because it substitutes beautifully for many grains in both sweet and savory dishes. However, quinoa is actually a seed that is rich in both protein and omega-3 fats.

- 1 teaspoon canola oil
- 3/4 cup uncooked quinoa
- 1/2 teaspoon nutmeg
- 1 cup water

- 1/2 cup vanilla almond milk
- 2 cups fresh blueberries
- 1 teaspoon vanilla

In a medium-sized heavy skillet, heat canola oil over medium-high heat. Add quinoa and nutmeg, and cook for 2 minutes, stirring frequently.

Add water and simmer uncovered for 10 minutes, or until quinoa is still slightly crunchy.

Add almond milk, blueberries, and vanilla, stirring well. Simmer for 4 minutes, ladle into bowls, and serve warm.

Makes 2 servings.

Calories: 185

Sodium: 17 mg

Bacon and Tomato Open-Faced Sandwiches

Though you may not want to eat it every morning, you can have low-sodium turkey bacon in moderation. This sandwich will satisfy your bacon-and-egg cravings beautifully without compromising your diet or your health.

- 4 slices low-sodium turkey bacon
- 2 slices whole-grain bread
- 1/2 teaspoon canola oil
- 4 large eggs
- 4 thin slices medium-ripe tomato
- 2 thin slices of reduced-fat Swiss cheese

Cook bacon in microwave according to package directions and set aside. Toast bread until lightly golden.

Heat canola oil in a medium-heavy skillet over medium heat, and add eggs. Cook for 1 minute to allow whites to begin setting, and then pierce yolks several times. Cook for about 5 minutes until yolks are cooked through. Remove eggs to a plate or cutting board, and add tomato slices to hot pan, off the heat, to warm.

Preheat oven to broil, and line a small baking sheet with foil. Place toast on foil, and add 2 tomato slices to each. Top each piece of toast with 2 eggs and 1 slice of cheese.

Broil for 1-2 minutes until cheese is bubbly. Serve hot.

Makes 2 servings.
Calories: 410
Sodium: 678 mg

Ranchero Tortilla Cups

If you have a taste for a south-of-the-border breakfast, this recipe will fit the bill. It looks like something you took a lot of care to prepare, but it actually takes just minutes. This recipe serves six, so it's a good one for weekend guests.

- 1 tablespoon olive oil, divided
- 6 (6-inch) flour tortillas
- 1/2 teaspoon salt substitute
- 1 (10-ounce) can unsalted black beans, rinsed and drained
- 3/4 cup low-sodium or homemade salsa

- 6 large eggs
- 1/2 cup part-skim shredded Mexican cheese
- 1/2 cup low-fat or nonfat sour cream
- Fresh parsley, chopped

Preheat oven to 375 degrees.

Using a pastry brush, lightly grease 6 cups of a jumbo muffin tin with some olive oil.

Use remaining olive oil to lightly coat one side of each tortilla, and sprinkle with salt substitute. Press each tortilla, oil side down, into a prepared muffin cup.

Layer black beans in each tortilla cup, followed by salsa. Then crack 1 egg into each, followed by shredded cheese.

Bake for about 15-17 minutes or until eggs are cooked through. Remove each cup to a plate, and top with a small dollop of sour cream. Garnish with parsley and serve.

Makes 6 servings.
Calories: 185
Sodium: 460 mg

Poached Eggs over Roasted Asparagus

This is a wonderful, light breakfast that is loaded with fresh flavor but won't weigh you down. Roasting brings out the sweet, nutty flavor of asparagus in a way that no other method of preparation can.

- 8 stalks fresh asparagus, trimmed and cut in half
- 1 teaspoon olive oil
- 1/2 teaspoon salt substitute
- 1/4 teaspoon freshly ground pepper
- 1/4 teaspoon freshly ground nutmeg
- 2 cups water
- 1 tablespoon white vinegar
- 4 large eggs
- 1/2 cup low-fat Swiss cheese, shredded

Preheat oven to 375 degrees.

Line a baking sheet with foil. Place asparagus on baking sheet, then toss with olive oil. Add salt, freshly ground pepper, and nutmeg evenly among asparagus spears. Bake for 10-12 minutes or just until slightly tender.

Meanwhile, bring water to a slow simmer in a medium saucepan. The water should have tiny bubbles around the edges and bottom without coming to an actual boil. Add vinegar, then crack eggs, 1 at a time, into a small bowl before gently pouring into simmering water. Cook for 3 minutes and then use a slotted spoon to remove eggs from water.

As soon as asparagus is done, divide 8 asparagus halves between 2 plates. Sprinkle each with half of the Swiss cheese, then top each with 2 eggs. Serve immediately.

Makes 2 servings.

Calories: 375

Sodium: 211 mg

Island Breakfast Smoothie

Even if you don't have time for a sit-down breakfast, you can still whip up a filling and nutritious smoothie in just seconds. This one makes just enough to fit into a 12-ounce travel mug, too.

- 1 (6-ounce) container of mango or peach Greek yogurt
- 1/4 cup low-fat milk
- 1/2 cup frozen mango chunks
- 3 tablespoons unsweetened coconut flakes
- 6 ice cubes

In a blender, combine yogurt, milk, mango, and coconut, and blend until well combined. Add ice cubes and blend until mango is well processed, and mixture is thick and creamy. Serve immediately.

Makes 1 large smoothie.

Calories: 220

Sodium: 90 mg

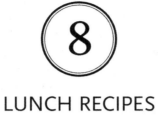

LUNCH RECIPES

Spinach Waldorf Salad

This crisp, refreshing salad combines the flavors of two classics, resulting in a crunchy, decadent dish that will make you rethink salads! The fat content may seem high, but don't worry; all of the fat in this salad comes from heart-healthful walnuts, avocados, and olive oil!

For the dressing:
- 1/4 cup nonfat Greek yogurt
- 1 tablespoon ripe avocado
- 1 tablespoon olive oil
- 1 teaspoon lemon juice
- 1/2 teaspoon scallions
- 1/2 teaspoon garlic, minced
- 1 teaspoon basil, minced
- 1 teaspoon parsley, minced

For the salad:
- 4 cups fresh spinach
- 1 cup apples, chopped
- 1/4 cup walnuts, chopped
- 2 slices low-sodium turkey bacon, crisped and chopped
- 1 tablespoon fresh scallions
- 1 tablespoon dried cranberries

To make the dressing:

Make the dressing first, and feel free to double the recipe if you'd like a heart-healthful dip or dressing for use with other meals. Start by combining yogurt, avocado, olive oil, and lemon juice in a small mixing bowl. Combine well, then add scallion, garlic, and herbs. Set aside.

To make the salad:

Toss salad ingredients together, and portion into 2-cup portions. Drizzle 1 tablespoon of dressing over each serving.

Makes about 2 (2-cup) servings.
Calories: 292
Sodium: 55 mg

"Going Greek" Chicken Tzatziki Wrap

Biting into this wrap is just as satisfying as hitting the fast-food restaurant. The fresh, crisp texture of the veggies and the creamy, mildly spicy zest of the sauce create a flavor profile that will thrill even the pickiest eaters.

For the dressing:
- 1/2 cup nonfat Greek yogurt
- 2 teaspoons fresh dill, chopped
- 1 tablespoon lemon juice
- 1 teaspoon chopped garlic
- 1/4 cup cucumber, diced

For the wraps:
- 4 whole-grain pitas
- 1 cup romaine lettuce, chopped
- 1/2 cup tomatoes, chopped
- 1/4 cup red onion, chopped
- 8 Kalamata olives, sliced
- 1/4 cup feta cheese

For the chicken:
- 2 boneless and skinless chicken breasts
- Olive oil cooking spray
- 1/2 teaspoon freshly ground pepper
- 1/2 teaspoon garlic powder
- 1/4 teaspoon oregano
- 1 teaspoon lemon juice

To make the dressing:

In a small mixing bowl, combine all of the ingredients for the dressing. Set aside while you cook the chicken.

To make the chicken:

Add chicken breast to a heated, heavy skillet coated with olive oil cooking spray. Sprinkle with freshly ground pepper, garlic, and oregano. Cook on medium-high heat for about 4-5 minutes on each side. Remove from skillet and drizzle with the lemon juice. Chop into bite-sized chunks.

To make the wraps:

Warm pitas in oven or microwave. Divide lettuce, tomatoes, red onions, and olives equally over each pita. Divide chicken evenly between 4 wraps, and sprinkle feta cheese over chicken. Drizzle 2 tablespoons of dressing over each pita. Fold each pita in half and serve.

Makes 4 servings.
Calories: 199
Sodium: 450 mg

Blackened Salmon Filet

Rich in heart-healthful omega-3s, salmon is quite possibly one of nature's perfect foods. Flaky and flavorful, this dish won't leave you feeling like you're on a diet. Pair with a crisp, green salad or grilled asparagus for a satisfying meal that will hold you through until dinner.

- 1 (6-ounce) salmon filet
- 1/4 teaspoon cayenne pepper
- 1/4 teaspoon freshly ground pepper
- 1/4 teaspoon salt substitute
- 1/2 teaspoon paprika
- 1/2 teaspoon garlic powder
- 1/4 teaspoon thyme
- 1/4 teaspoon dried Italian seasoning
- Olive oil cooking spray

Rinse salmon and pat dry. Combine all spices and rub on both sides of salmon. Let rest for 10 minutes. Spray a medium-sized heavy skillet with olive oil cooking spray, and heat over medium-high heat.

Add salmon to center of skillet, and cook for about 3 minutes per side. Test for doneness. It's cooked through when flaky and opaque. If you'd like it a little more well done, cook it a bit longer, testing it once per minute.

Makes 1 serving.

Calories: 288

Sodium: 151 mg

Grilled Coconut Shrimp

Shrimp is an excellent source of protein and potassium. Reminiscent of sun-kissed days and sand between your toes, this recipe will make you feel like you're on vacation. Serve with a fruit salad and some brown rice.

- 12 jumbo shrimp
- 1/2 cup unsweetened coconut milk
- 1/2 teaspoon paprika (smoked is best)

- 12 cherry tomatoes
- 12 fresh 1-inch cubes of pineapple
- 2 green sweet peppers, each sliced into 6 strips (12 total)

Soak peeled, deveined shrimp in unsweetened coconut milk overnight, or for at least 30 minutes. Remove and pat dry with a paper towel, then sprinkle with paprika.

Using metal or bamboo kabob skewers, thread shrimp, tomatoes, pineapple, and peppers in an alternating pattern, using 3 of each per skewer.

Grill or oven broil until each shrimp turns pink and curls into a "C" shape about 6-8 minutes.

Remove from heat and serve immediately.

Makes 4 servings.
Calories: 74
Sodium: 34 mg

Ooey-Gooey Tuna Melt

When nothing but a deli-style sandwich will satisfy, this one delivers all the flavor and texture, without the high fat and salt content of most deli lunches.

- 1 (5-ounce) can chunk light tuna, packed in water and drained
- 1 tablespoon Dijon mustard
- 1 tablespoon reduced-fat sour cream
- 1 teaspoon dried dill
- 1/4 teaspoon paprika
- 1 tablespoon celery, diced
- 1/4 teaspoon freshly ground pepper
- 4 slices whole-grain bread
- 2 thin slices reduced-fat Swiss cheese
- 4 thin slices red onion
- 4 large lettuce leaves
- 1 green pepper, sliced into slivers

Preheat oven to low broil.

In a small mixing bowl, combine tuna, mustard, sour cream, dill, paprika, celery, and freshly ground pepper. Place 2 slices of whole grain bread on a baking sheet, and put half of the tuna mixture on each slice.

Add one slice of cheese to each sandwich, and place under broiler for about 2 minutes or until cheese melts. Remove from oven and layer onion, lettuce, and green pepper onto each sandwich.

Top with second slice of bread, and enjoy with a pickle wedge.

Makes 2 servings.
Calories: 269
Sodium: 408 mg

Grilled Chicken and Veggies

This is a great lunch for those weekdays when you're in a hurry. You can prepare the chicken and veggies in advance and toss them into a to-go container for a tasty, healthful lunch in a pinch.

- 1/2 teaspoon olive oil
- 1 (6-ounce) chicken breast
- 1/2 teaspoon salt substitute, divided
- 1/2 teaspoon garlic powder
- 1/2 teaspoon paprika
- 1/2 teaspoon Italian seasoning
- 1 green pepper, sliced
- 10 cherry tomatoes
- 1/2 cup broccoli
- 1/2 cup red onions, sliced
- 1/2 cup zucchini, cubed

Heat olive oil in a medium-sized heavy skillet on medium-high heat. Sprinkle chicken breast with half of the salt, garlic powder, and paprika, and add to skillet. Let chicken cook on one side for 3 minutes, then flip and add remaining seasoning. Add veggies and cover. Cook for another 3-4 minutes.

Makes 1 serving.

Calories: 385

Sodium: 147 mg

Spinach and Chicken Salad

Forget about that chef's salad or same old iceberg lettuce. This fresh salad will satisfy you for the entire afternoon, and the slightly exotic flavor is a nice change of pace. As a bonus, each serving contains over 900 mg of potassium.

- 1 teaspoon olive oil
- 2 (6-ounce) chicken breasts
- 1/2 teaspoon mild curry powder
- 2 cups fresh baby spinach leaves
- 12 cherry tomatoes
- 1 small red onion, sliced thinly
- 1 small yellow pepper, diced
- 2 tablespoons low-sodium vinaigrette

Heat olive oil in a heavy skillet over medium-high heat. Sprinkle breasts with curry powder on both sides, and sauté for 5-7 minutes on each side.

Combine spinach leaves, tomatoes, onion, and pepper in a large bowl, and add vinaigrette. Pile onto 2 salad plates. Slice chicken breast into strips, and serve on top of salad.

Makes 2 servings.

Calories: 315

Sodium: 285 mg

Garlicky Tomato Soup

This creamy soup far surpasses the canned variety and takes less than thirty minutes to prepare. Served with a crusty roll and a fresh green salad, it's a light but delicious lunch dish. It's also got a whopping 1,237 mg of potassium per serving.

- 1 teaspoon olive oil
- 2 cloves fresh garlic, crushed
- 1/4 cup sweet white onion, chopped
- 1/2 teaspoon salt substitute
- 1/4 teaspoon freshly ground pepper
- 1 teaspoon granulated sugar
- 1 (6-ounce) can low-sodium tomato paste
- 1 1/2 cups reduced-fat milk

In a medium-sized skillet, heat olive oil over medium-low heat. Add garlic and onion, and sauté just until onion is translucent, about 5-6 minutes.

Add salt substitute, freshly ground pepper, and sugar, and stir well, then add tomato paste. Stir with a whisk or fork to blend well, then add milk and whisk until well blended.

Turn heat to low and simmer for 15 minutes. Pour into mugs or bowls to serve.

Makes 2 servings.
Calories: 165
Sodium: 367 mg

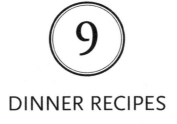

DINNER RECIPES

Beef Tostadas

Easy to make and fun to eat, this recipe combines the best of Tex-Mex flavors without all of the sodium and fat that restaurant meals typically include. Serve with a fresh, green salad for a light, summer meal.

- 1 tablespoon olive oil
- 1/2 pound ground turkey
- 1/2 teaspoon cumin
- 1/2 teaspoon freshly ground pepper
- 1/2 teaspoon chili powder
- 1 (3-ounce) can low-sodium tomato paste

- 1 can nonfat black beans
- 4 crispy tostada shells
- 2 cups Mexican cheese, shredded
- 2 cups lettuce, shredded
- 2 cups fresh tomato, chopped
- 3/4 cup white onion, diced
- 3/4 cup black olives, sliced

Lightly coat heavy skillet in olive oil. Brown the ground turkey in a heavy skillet over medium-high heat. Season turkey with cumin, freshly ground pepper, and chili powder. Cook for 10 minutes until turkey is completely cooked through, then add tomato paste and black beans, stirring well. Reduce heat to low and cover to keep warm.

Place one tostada shell on each plate, and top with one-quarter of the turkey mixture. Top with shredded cheese, then lettuce, tomato, onion, and olives.

Makes 4 servings.
Calories: 278
Sodium: 620 mg

Ginger-Spiced Haddock Filets

Rich in omega-3 fats, haddock is a firm, moist fish that takes flavors well. You may also substitute cod or flounder if haddock isn't available.

- 2 tablespoons olive oil, divided
- 1 teaspoon Dijon mustard
- 2 teaspoons fresh ginger, grated
- 2 teaspoons honey
- 1 tablespoon rice vinegar
- 2 teaspoons low-sodium soy sauce
- 1/4 cup orange juice
- 4 (6-ounce) haddock filets
- 1 cup scallions, chopped
- 10 cherry tomatoes, halved

In a small bowl, combine 1 tablespoon olive oil, mustard, ginger, honey, vinegar, soy sauce, and orange juice. Add fish filets and cover. Allow to marinate in refrigerator for 1 hour.

Heat a large, heavy skillet on medium-high heat. Add remaining olive oil and heat for 1 minute. Add fish filets (reserving marinade), then arrange the scallions and tomato around edges of the pan. Cook for 1 minute.

Turn the fish over, turn heat to low, and pour marinade over all. Cook covered for 3 minutes.

Serve haddock with vegetables and sauce ladled on top.

Makes 4 servings.
Calories: 368
Sodium: 427 mg

Lemon-Thyme Chicken Breasts

This quick chicken dish is light and filled with the flavors of summer. With a green salad or some steamed asparagus, it's sure to become one of your favorite go-to meals.

- 4 (6-ounce) boneless chicken breasts
- 1 teaspoon olive oil
- 1/2 teaspoon salt substitute
- 1/2 teaspoon freshly ground pepper
- 2 tablespoons fresh thyme, stems removed and chopped
- 2 teaspoons lemon zest
- Juice of 1 large lemon

Pound chicken breasts with the heels of your hand or a rolling pin until uniform thickness.

Rub each breast with olive oil on both sides, then season with salt substitute and freshly ground pepper.

Heat a large, heavy skillet on medium-high heat, and add chicken breasts. Sauté for 4 minutes, then turn. Add thyme and lemon zest, cover, and cook for another 4-6 minutes until chicken is done. Squeeze lemon juice over breasts before serving.

Makes 4 servings.
Calories: 330
Sodium: 148 mg

Cheesy Vegetarian Rice Casserole

This vegetarian casserole delivers on pure comfort and heartwarming flavor. It's a great dish to make ahead on the weekend and refrigerate for a busy weeknight dinner.

- 2 cups fresh broccoli, chopped
- 1 cup fresh spinach, chopped
- 1 cup fresh cauliflower, chopped
- 1/2 cup fresh carrots, diced
- 1/2 cup red bell peppers, diced
- 1/2 teaspoon salt substitute
- 1/4 teaspoon freshly ground pepper
- 1 teaspoon paprika
- 1/2 cup reduced-fat Swiss cheese, shredded
- 3/4 cup medium-grain brown rice
- 1 cup unflavored almond milk
- 1/2 cup plain low-fat yogurt

Preheat oven to 375 degrees.

Combine vegetables in a large mixing bowl. Add salt substitute, freshly ground pepper, and paprika, and toss well with your hands to distribute evenly.

Add shredded cheese and rice, and toss again to combine. Pour into a 9 x 13–inch glass casserole dish. In a small bowl, mix together almond milk and yogurt, and pour over casserole.

Bake for 50 minutes or until rice is tender.

Makes 4 servings as an entrée or 8 servings as a side dish.

Calories: 412

Sodium: 346 mg

Citrus-Kissed Fish in Foil

This is a wonderful way to cook delicious fish with no muss and no fuss. The orange and lime add just the right amount of freshness, and there's no pan to wash when you're done. You'll also get a healthful 640 mg of potassium.

- 4 (6-ounce) flounder filets
- 1 teaspoon olive oil
- 1/2 teaspoon salt substitute
- 1/2 teaspoon freshly ground pepper
- 8 thin slices of orange
- 8 thin slices of lime
- 4 sprigs fresh rosemary
- Juice of one orange
- Juice of one small lime
- 1/2 cup dry white wine

Preheat oven to 400 degrees.

Cut 4 (12-inch) lengths of aluminum foil and lay out on counter.

Rub each fish filet with olive oil, and season both sides with salt substitute and freshly ground pepper. Place each filet on one sheet of foil. Alternate slices of orange and lime on each filet, allocating 2 of each fruit per filet.

Lay rosemary sprigs on top of fruit slices, and squeeze both orange and lime juice over each filet. Pour 1/4 of the wine over the first filet, quickly fold edges of foil up at ends, and pull sides together at top before rolling a couple of times to seal. Make sure to leave about 3-4 inches of "headroom" for the fish.

Repeat with the remaining packets, and place all 4 packets onto a lipped cookie sheet or large baking pan.

Bake for 20 minutes, place each packet on a plate, and allow your guests to cut the packets open at the table.

Makes 4 servings.
Calories: 230
Sodium: 180 mg

Fruited Pork Loin

The combination of succulent pork and sweet fruit has long been a classic. This recipe uses fresh herbs and orange zest to give the dish a light and refreshing taste.

- 1 pound pork tenderloin, unseasoned
- 1/2 cup unsweetened dried cranberries
- 1/2 cup dried apricots
- 1 cup water
- 1 cup Marsala wine
- 1 teaspoon fresh sage, chopped
- 1 teaspoon fresh tarragon, chopped
- 1/2 teaspoon salt substitute
- 1/2 teaspoon freshly ground pepper
- 1 teaspoon orange zest

Preheat oven to 375 degrees.

Line a baking pan with foil. Place tenderloin onto the foil, and arrange cranberries and apricots around meat.

Pour water and Marsala wine over all, then season with sage, tarragon, salt substitute, and freshly ground pepper, turning meat once to coat evenly.

Sprinkle orange zest over tenderloin, cover with foil, and bake for 45-50 minutes, uncovering the dish for final 10 minutes.

Allow meat to sit for 10 minutes before slicing, and arrange on a platter with fruit ladled over the top.

Makes 4 servings.
Calories: 250
Sodium: 25 mg

Herbed Turkey Medallions with Rice

This dish is quick to prepare and is great for planned leftovers. Make an extra batch to pack for a healthful brown-bag lunch. If turkey breast is unavailable, substitute sliced turkey thigh.

- 1 teaspoon olive oil
- 4 (6-ounce) turkey breast cutlets
- 1 cup yellow onion, sliced thinly
- 1 tablespoon fresh sage, chopped
- 1 tablespoon fresh rosemary
- 1/2 teaspoon freshly ground pepper
- 1 cup low-sodium chicken broth
- 2 cups short-grain brown rice
- 4 cups water
- 1 tablespoon cornstarch
- 1/2 cup dry white wine

In a large heavy skillet, heat olive oil on medium-high heat.

Brown the turkey for about 5 minutes on each side, and then add onion, sage, rosemary, freshly ground pepper, and chicken broth.

Meanwhile, combine rice and water in a large casserole, cover, and microwave on high for 20 minutes.

In a small bowl, stir cornstarch into wine until smooth, then whisk into broth. Reduce heat to low, and simmer for 15-20 minutes. Serve over rice.

Makes 4 servings.

Calories: 205

Sodium: 120 mg

Asian-Style Chicken Skewers

These simple and quick-cooking chicken skewers are similar to what you'd find at your favorite Asian restaurant. Children love them, so they're a great dish to make for youngest family members.

- 2 cloves garlic, crushed
- 1 teaspoon fresh ginger, grated
- 1/4 cup low-sodium soy sauce
- 1/2 teaspoon red pepper flakes
- 12 (2-ounce) boneless and skinless chicken thighs
- 4 scallions, finely chopped
- 6 bamboo skewers

Combine garlic, ginger, soy sauce, and red pepper flakes in a large plastic bag.

Cut each thigh in half lengthwise, and add all to plastic bag. Place on a plate and marinate in refrigerator for a minimum of 2 hours. Meanwhile, soak 6 bamboo skewers in water for 30 minutes.

Preheat oven to 400 degrees.

Remove each chicken thigh from the bag, tapping to remove excess marinade, and thread 2 halves lengthwise onto each skewer. Place onto foil-lined baking pan, and bake for 20 minutes or until chicken is done.

Garnish with scallions and serve over cooked rice, rice noodles, or with sautéed vegetables.

Makes 6 servings.
Calories: 167
Sodium: 310 mg

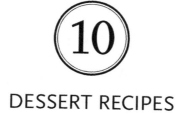

DESSERT RECIPES

Baked Spiced Apples

This dessert is a wonderful end to a fall or winter meal, or anytime you'd like something warm and comforting. This recipe also works well with firm pears such as Bosc.

- 4 firm apples, such as Cortland or Granny Smith, peeled and cored
- 3 teaspoons light brown sugar
- 1/2 teaspoon cinnamon
- 1/2 teaspoon cardamom
- 1 cup unsweetened apple cider
- 1 cup unsweetened orange juice
- 1 tablespoon cornstarch
- 2 tablespoons cold water
- 2 tablespoons chopped black walnuts

Preheat oven to 350 degrees.

Place apples in a lined baking pan, and sprinkle with brown sugar, cinnamon, and cardamom.

Pour cider and orange juice into the dish and bake for 20-25 minutes. Remove apples to 4 dessert dishes and set aside.

Pour baking juices into a small saucepan, and heat on medium heat to a low simmer. In a separate bowl, mix cornstarch and water, then whisk into pan. Continue stirring until thickened, then spoon over each apple. Sprinkle chopped walnuts over each portion and serve warm.

Makes 4 servings.

Calories: 143

Sodium: 3 mg

Easy Peach Sorbet

A sweet, fresh-tasting, frozen treat is at your fingertips, even on a busy weeknight. This refreshing dessert takes just a minute to prepare and about 90 minutes to freeze. Change it up with seasonal fruits, such as watermelon, pears, and cantaloupe.

- 2 cups fresh or frozen peaches, peeled and sliced
- 1/4 cup orange juice
- 1 teaspoon almond extract
- 1 teaspoon granulated sugar

In a blender, combine peaches, orange juice, almond extract, and sugar, and blend on high until smooth. Spoon into 2 dessert dishes, and freeze until slightly slushy. Stir gently, freeze for 1 more hour, and serve.

Makes 2 servings.

Calories: 105

Sodium: 0.5 mg

Raspberry Walnut Sorbet

This creamy, delicious dessert is high in antioxidants from the black walnuts and fresh raspberries. Meanwhile, the agave nectar provides a low-glycemic alternative to sugar without using artificial sweeteners.

- 2 cups fresh ripe raspberries
- 1/4 cup walnuts, chopped
- 1 teaspoon lemon juice
- 2 tablespoons organic agave nectar

In a food processor or blender, puree all ingredients together. Freeze in an ice cream maker. Alternately, spread fruit mixture onto a cookie sheet and place in freezer.

Every 20 minutes, scrape through fruit mixture with a spoon so that it doesn't freeze into a solid mass—this will keep it nice and light.

Makes 4 servings.

Calories: 109

Sodium: 0.2 mg

Pumpkin Vanilla Pudding

This decadent dessert will make you think that you're cheating on your diet when, in fact, you're not. Sure to please your sweet tooth, this pudding delivers fiber, antioxidants, and beta carotene. This smooth, luscious dessert is equally tasty served warm or cold.

- 1 1/2 cups fat-free vanilla yogurt
- 1 (20-ounce) can plain pumpkin puree
- 1/2 teaspoon ground nutmeg
- 1/2 teaspoon ground cinnamon
- 1 vanilla bean

Combine yogurt, pumpkin puree, nutmeg, and cinnamon in a medium-sized mixing bowl. Scrape vanilla beans out of husk and into mixture. Mix well until all ingredients are combined. Chill until ready to serve.

Makes 6 servings.

Calories: 67

Sodium: 38 mg

Creamy Greek Fruit Salad

If you like light, fruity desserts with just a touch of sweetness, you're going to love this salad. It's refreshing yet satisfying and great for the warmer seasons.

- 6 mint leaves
- 1 tablespoon honey
- 1/2 cup plain Greek yogurt
- 1 cup apples, cubed
- 1 cup red seedless grapes, halved
- 1/4 cup pecans, chopped
- 1 cup mango, cubed

Crush the mint leaves in a medium-sized mixing bowl. Add the honey and yogurt, stirring until smooth. Add the apples, grapes, pecans, and mango, and toss gently to coat.

Makes 4 servings.

Calories: 149

Sodium: 24 mg

Tropical Chocolate Meringue Puffs

Two secrets behind the success of this recipe are to make sure your egg whites are room temperature and your cream of tartar is fresh. If you forget to take your eggs out of the fridge early enough, just place the whole, unshelled eggs in a bowl of warm water for a few minutes while you gather the rest of the ingredients. The orange extract adds an exotic twist to these much-loved chocolate meringue puff cookies, but if you'd rather take the traditional route, simply replace the orange extract with an equal amount of vanilla.

- 3 medium egg whites
- 1/2 teaspoon cream of tartar
- 1/2 cup sugar
- 1/2 teaspoon orange extract
- 1 1/2 tablespoons cocoa powder
- 6 ounces bittersweet chocolate, melted but not hot
- Olive oil cooking spray

Preheat oven to 350 degrees.

In a dry, medium-sized glass bowl, beat egg whites and cream of tartar with a hand mixer on medium speed until peaks begin to form, about 1 minute. Add sugar slowly while you continue to mix.

Add orange extract and continue beating, scraping sides of bowl frequently, until mixture forms firm peaks and is glossy.

In a separate bowl, stir cocoa into melted chocolate, then gently fold mixture into meringue. Line baking sheets with parchment paper, then apply olive oil cooking spray. Drop rounded spoonfuls of mixture onto parchment paper.

Bake on middle rack for 8-12 minutes until puffs are firm on outside but still soft on inside. You may want to switch to the top rack for the last couple of minutes so that the bottoms don't brown. When puffs are cool, remove from parchment paper, and store in an airtight container for up to 1 week.

Makes about 3 dozen cookies. Serving size equals 2 cookies.

Calories: 72

Sodium: 9 mg

Nutty Peach Yogurt Shake

This healthful take on a traditional favorite may just become your new favorite drink. The almond milk adds magnesium and lends a silky, nutty flavor. Add in the potassium from the banana, and you've got a great post-workout drink or after-dinner dessert.

- 1 cup ice
- 1 1/2 cups almond milk
- 1 cup vanilla Greek yogurt
- 2 fresh ripe peaches, peeled, pitted, and chopped
- 1 large ripe banana, peeled

Combine ice, milk, and yogurt in a blender, then add fruit. Blend on low speed until fruit and ice are roughly incorporated into the mixture, then on high for about 20 seconds until smooth and creamy.

Makes 3 (12-ounce) servings.

Calories: 213

Sodium: 206 mg

Chocolate Strawberry Mousse

Everybody needs to indulge sometimes, but with this dessert, you're getting the chocolate you crave without the guilt.

- 1 1/2 teaspoons unflavored gelatin
- 1/4 cup hot water
- 1 tablespoon cocoa powder
- 3 eggs, separated and room temperature
- 1/8 teaspoon cream of tartar
- 1/4 cup superfine sugar
- 1/2 cup fresh, ripe strawberries, sliced
- 1 tablespoon honey
- 1/2 teaspoon lemon zest

Stir the gelatin into hot water until dissolved, then add cocoa.

In a medium-sized mixing bowl, combine egg whites and cream of tartar. Beat with hand mixer until soft peaks form, about 1 minute. Slowly add sugar, and beat on high until stiff peaks form and mixture is glossy. Continue beating on high, and add egg yolks 1 at a time until well combined.

Add gelatin mixture slowly as you continue beating on high until you have a nice, smooth mousse, about 30 seconds to 1 minute.

Divide into separate serving ramekins and refrigerate.

In a separate small bowl, toss strawberries with honey and lemon zest. Refrigerate until you're ready to serve.

Top each mousse with a tablespoon of strawberry mixture and serve.

Makes 4 servings.

Calories: 92

Sodium: 18 mg

SEVEN-DAY DASH DIET MEAL PLAN

Here you'll find seven days of menu ideas to help you get started on your DASH diet. If you opt to follow them, they'll help you get accustomed to healthier portions and also introduce you to some new flavors and dishes.

If you want to continue using the menu plan after the first week, simply mix and match your favorite meals in subsequent weeks. Just keep an eye on the calories, fat, and sodium of the recipes you choose, so that you can adjust other meals if needed.

The following menu plans are for a 2,000 calorie diet, allowing 1,500 mg of sodium daily. The actual menus run between 1,700-1,800 calories to allow for extra snacks of fruit, extra helpings of veggies, or an extra beverage of milk or juice.

If you need to adjust the calories up or down, remember to follow these tips:

- If you need to lower your calories, decrease your servings of grains and fruits by one or two each.
- If you need to raise your calorie intake, increase your fruits and vegetables first, then grains.

If you don't need to keep the sodium intake to a lower level, you can be more liberal with table salt and use more condiments, such as teriyaki sauce or prepared salad dressings.

The only beverages specified on the menu plans are milk and juice. You're free to have water, sweetened or unsweetened hot tea, or coffee at every meal. If you have more leeway in your calories, feel free to add fruit juice or milk to a meal.

Note: Dishes marked with a star (*) are provided in the recipe section.

Day 1

Breakfast:

2 scrambled eggs
1/2 cup cantaloupe
1 slice whole-wheat toast with jam
8 ounces skim or 1 percent milk

Snack:

1 Chewy Cranberry-Apricot Bar*
Small glass of milk

Lunch:

Spinach-Waldorf Salad*
1 medium orange

Dinner:

Lemon-Thyme Chicken Breast*
1 cup oven-roasted carrots
1 whole-grain roll

Dessert:

1 cup watermelon

Day 2

Breakfast:

 1 cup cantaloupe and apple chunks
 1/2 cup cottage cheese

Snack:

 10 low-sodium crackers
 4 ounces part-skim cheese
 1 medium pear

Lunch:

 Ooey-Gooey Tuna Melt*
 1/2 cup sliced strawberries

Dinner:

 1 filet broiled cod or other fish
 1 cup steamed spinach
 1/2 baked sweet potato with margarine or salt substitute
 1 cup brown rice

Dessert:

 Easy Peach Sorbet*

Day 3

Breakfast:

1/2 cup whole-grain cereal, such as Wheaties or Uncle Sam
1/4 cup skim or 1 percent milk
1/2 cup strawberries
1 medium banana

Snack:

1 sliced tomato with low-sodium salad dressing
1 stick string cheese

Lunch:

1 cup vegetable soup
Salad with spring greens and red onion
1 tablespoon low-sodium dressing

Dinner:

Citrus-Kissed Fish in Foil*
1 cup green beans with 1 teaspoon margarine or olive oil
1 cup steamed quinoa with olive oil and pepper

Dessert:

1 frozen fudge pop

Day 4

Breakfast:

> Toasted Oat and Fruit Parfait*
> 6 ounces orange juice

Snack:

> 1/2 cup cottage cheese
> 1/2 cup peaches

Lunch:

> Garlicky Tomato Soup*
> 1 small, whole-grain roll
> 1 medium apple

Dinner:

> Fruited Pork Loin*
> 1 cup brown rice
> 1 cup sautéed spinach

Dessert:

> 1 nonfat pudding cup

Day 5

Breakfast:

> Better-Than-a-Latte Smoothie*
> 1 medium apple

Snack:

> 1 part-skim mozzarella stick
> 1/4 cup sunflower seeds (unsalted)

Lunch:

> 1 cup low-sodium barley soup
> 10 low-sodium crackers
> 1 medium banana

Dinner:

> Asian-Style Chicken Skewers*
> 1 cup sautéed kale with olive oil and salt substitute
> 1 cup roasted carrots with olive oil and salt substitute
> 1/2 cup brown rice

Dessert:

> 1 large slice honeydew melon

Day 6

Breakfast:

Bacon and Tomato Open-Faced Sandwich*
1/2 cup sliced pears

Snack:

1 cup Crispy Kale Chips*
1 medium orange

Lunch:

Chicken breast sandwich on whole-wheat pita with 2 slices tomato,
sliced onion, and 1/2 cup lettuce
1 tablespoon low-fat mayonnaise
1 medium banana

Dinner:

1 filet baked salmon
1 cup steamed cauliflower with 1 teaspoon margarine or olive oil
1/2 cup sautéed mushrooms and onions
6 spears roasted asparagus with olive oil and pepper

Dessert:

Baked Spiced Apple*

Day 7

Breakfast:

Island Breakfast Smoothie*
1/4 cup almonds

Snack:

1 (6-ounce) container Greek yogurt, any flavor
1 cup watermelon chunks

Lunch:

Salad with 6 shrimp, 1 cup romaine, 1/2 cup tomato,
and 1/2 cup red pepper
1 tablespoon balsamic vinaigrette
1 slice whole-wheat toast with margarine

Dinner:

Ranchero Tortilla Cups*
1 cup mixed, fresh fruit

Dessert:

1 (1-ounce) square dark chocolate

CONCLUSION

You now have everything you need to get a great start on a healthful new lifestyle through the DASH diet.

Read through the tips sections whenever you feel as though you need a quick pick-me-up. Be sure to set small goals that come with equally small but pleasurable rewards. This will help you stay motivated as you work toward your weight-loss and health objectives.

Visit farmer's markets, cooking demonstrations, and other places where you can find new ideas for healthful meals to add to your DASH repertoire, and don't be afraid to try new things.

Losing weight, lowering your blood pressure, and overhauling your overall health takes commitment, but it should be an exciting and empowering time for you.

REFERENCES

American Heart Association (2012, April 4). "Managing Blood Pressure with a Heart-Healthy Diet." Retrieved January 20, 2013, from Heart.org: http://www.heart.org/HEARTORG/Conditions/HighBloodPressure/ PreventionTreatmentofHighBloodPressure/Managing-Blood-Pressure-with-a-Heart-Healthy-Diet_UCM_301879_Article.jsp

"Liese AD, Nichols M, Sun X, D'Agostino RB Jr, Haffner SM (2009)." "Adherence to the DASH Diet Is Inversely Associated with Incidence of Type 2 Diabetes: The Insulin Resistance Atherosclerosis Study." *Diabetes Care.*

Nelson JA, Zeratsky KA (2010, April). "DASH Diet: Healthy Eating to Lower Your Blood Pressure." Retrieved January 19, 2013, from MayoClinic.com: http://www.MayoClinic.com/health/dash-diet/HI00047

Made in the USA
Middletown, DE
02 November 2019